Hawaiian Sandalwood Essential Oil

Benefits, Properties, Applications, Studies & Recipes

by Ann Sullivan

Published in USA by:

Ann Sullivan
217 N. Seacrest Blvd #9
Boynton Beach
FL 33425

© Copyright 2017

ISBN-13: ISBN-13: 978-1548243234
ISBN-10: 154824323X

Table of Contents

Introduction

What are essential oils, and how might they be used for therapeutic purposes?

Essential oils are ultra-potent oils, extracted from plants and flowers that have been utilized in medicine for centuries. Presently, they're most commonly used to supplement pharmaceutical medication, but they can also be an effective alternative to pharmaceuticals if you don't have access to them. Before you dismiss essential oils to support the body's natural defenses against injuries and illness, look at the historical evidence of the oils' therapeutic competence in practice. Your average age-old medical text will demonstrate that essential oils, herbs, and plenty of other natural ingredients have, for thousands of years, successfully enhanced immune function to meet and defeat any number of ailments and injuries. Though traditional medicine is considered "alternative" now, it was once the gold standard. And, frankly, perhaps it still should be, as these natural age-tested remedies can fortify the body's battlements against everything from simple maladies, like headaches, cuts and bruises, to serious diseases, like cancer.

Essential oils are deemed "essential," because the oils are composed of the "essence" of the plant. The difference between essential oils and other oils – like olive oil or vegetable oil, for instance – is that essential oils have high volatility and reduced fixation, which results in faster evaporation, enabling their popular use in aromatherapy.

Even at high temperatures, olive and vegetable oils don't evaporate.

Essential oils are especially necessary when it comes to a major natural or man-made disaster or some potential viral outbreak. In these types of dire situations, you may not have quick access (or any access at all) to your standard pharmaceutical supply; so, essential oils, along with other alternative medicines, will be your go-to wellness aids in the case of social collapse, viral outbreak or devastating natural disaster. When medical access is null and void, alternatives to our modern-day standard are the only chance we have to keep pathogens at bay.

You probably don't realize that you already use essential oils every day. They're in perfumes, shampoos, soaps, ointments...they're even used in furniture polish. Why are they found in so many aromatic products? Well, basically, because essential oils are super concentrated aromatic liquids, so their scent is remarkably strong. Let's put this into perspective: to steam tea, you use a few leaves of peppermint or juniper; to produce a single ounce of essential oil, five whole *pounds* of peppermint or juniper leaves are required. Some sources claim that to produce twelve pounds of essential oil would necessitate an acre of peppermint, juniper, or any other oil you're looking to produce en masse. Unlike vegetable oil, you don't often find concentrated therapeutic-grade essential oils sold in bulk; instead the oils are often sold in easily carried small, dark bottles, perfect for your GOOD bag (Get Out Of Dodge). Which is exactly what this book is aiming to help you do –

get out of dodge with your most vital of essential oils intact, a good supply of sandalwood essential oil.

Why sandalwood, you ask? Well, to get you quickly up to speed on this most essential of oils, below we've provided a condensed synopsis of sandalwood, after which we'll outline in greater detail the oil's history, properties, and common therapeutic uses, so that you – the consumer – might have a better understanding of the oil's benefits and applications. We've even provided supportive remedies for pure sandalwood, as well as blended recipes that incorporate the valuable oil. Chapter 3 will further detail past scientific research on sandalwood essential oil.

Now, let's get down to it.

Essential Oil 101: the Basics of Sandalwood

Summary: Hawaiian Sandalwood, or Santalum paniculatum, has traditional spiritual and cultural uses. For hundreds of years, Ayurvedic medicine has used sandalwood to treat inflammation and infection. The soothing nature of sandalwood has also prompted uses as an anti-depressant and relaxant. This is due to sandalwood's high volume of sesquiterpenes, which stimulate the brain's pineal gland which, in turn, calms the nervous system by producing melatonin, a strong antioxidant, in the blood stream. This benefits both the user's sleep cycle and the immune system. Cultivated in India, sandalwood has also recently been shown to combat several cancers, including cervical, prostate, breast and skin cancers, according to studies done by Brigham Young University.

Description: Sandalwood oil is commonly extracted through steam distillation. The wood is most often used. The oil is clear yellow in color, medium-thick in consistency, and has a medium rich woodsy floral scent.

Uses: Beyond those applications previously mentioned, additional uses for Sandalwood essential oil include supporting the body's defenses against skin issues, dermatitis, acne, dry skin, oily skin, stretch marks, scars, sensitive skin, wrinkles, cold sores, herpes simplex, candida, chapped skin, laryngitis, colds, flu, asthma, cough, throat infections, bronchitis, yeast infections, leucorrhea, hemorrhoids, impotence, diarrhea, urinary tract infections, sleep disorders, and cancer. Sandalwood also strengthens the immune system. When it comes to the mind, the oil calms and relaxes, which is helpful when easing stress or anxiety.

Properties: Antioxidant, anti-inflammatory, antibacterial, antiviral, antifungal, antiseptic, antispasmodic, antidepressant, aphrodisiac, astringent, sedative, diuretic, hypotensive, carminative, expectorant, digestive, tonic, and stimulant.

Application: Apply neat or undiluted. You can apply topically, inhale directly, diffuse or use as a dietary supplement.

Safety Precautions: Sandalwood oil is generally regarded as safe (GRAS). There is no need to dilute, and those with sensitive skin can use this oil safely. If pregnant or breastfeeding, always consult with your physician when using essential oils.

Fun facts: Sandalwood comes from the heartwood of the evergreen tree, which is native to southern Asia. Applications for sandalwood date back thousands of years to the De Materia Medica, a standard reference text which recorded hundreds of treatments. Dioscorides documented sandalwood's therapeutic uses in this book in 78 AD, and these references were used all the way up to the seventeenth century. Sandalwood was also used in embalming practices during funeral services to aid in the soul's transmigration.

Chapter 1 – Benefits of Sandalwood Essential Oil

Sandalwood essential oil offers several therapeutic benefits; but you may be wondering what these benefits are. In this chapter, we'll take a closer look at the history of sandalwood and its many uses.

Cultivation of Sandalwood

Sandalwood is an aromatic wood from the genera, Santalum. In this book, we will be covering the species, Santalum paniculatum which is commonly used in the making of essential oils. Generally, Santalum genus woods are yellow, heavy, slow-growing, hold their scent for dozens of years, and grow to medium heights. They are related to the same family as mistletoe. Sandalwood, in its various species, are found in Hawaii, Pacific Islands, Nepal, India, Bangladesh, Sri Lanka, Pakistan, and Australia. Hawaiian

Sandalwood was amongst three exported sandalwood species in the decades between 1790 and 1825. This shrank the supply of Hawaiian Sandalwood, but it has made a comeback in recent years. Unlike most oils, sandalwood is harvested through use of the entire tree, including the roots and the stump, which is why it is one of the more expensive oils.

A History of Sandalwood

Sandalwood, and the oil extracted from it, is highly and pleasantly fragranced. Being as such, both have been valued for hundreds of years and have thereby been overharvested, leading to threatened species, like that of Santalum album in South India.

The wood is so popular and valued in these regions that it is used in many Hindu rituals and ceremonies. For instance, a paste is made from sandalwood and is used to decorate icons and religious utensils, as well as to anoint the foreheads, chests, or necks of worshippers. Only the pure may prepare this paste, thus priests often prepare it in the temples during the ceremony by hand-grinding the wood atop a granite slab, slowly adding water as it's ground. The thick paste is then combined with saffron and pigments. One area, Tirupati, applies the sandalwood paste to the skin to protect it. In fact, in Ayurveda and Hinduism, sandalwood draws one nearer to the divine and is thereby considered one of the most holy elements.

Hinduism is not the only religion to celebrate

sandalwood. Buddhism and Islam, as well, consider sandalwood holy. In Buddhism, sandalwood is one of the lotus groups. It is noted in a variety of Pāli Canon suttas and is used in meditation to keep the meditator aware and present, while also transforming his or her desires. In Islam, the paste is applied as a sign of devotion in Sufi tradition to the grave of a Sufi. In the 19th century, some areas of India would anoint the Prophet Mohammed's symbolic footprints in sandalwood paste. Sandalwood was even seen as so powerful that it might rid of an epidemic. In these cases, an imprint of a hand was prepared with sandalwood paste, and this was paraded through town so that the sick might be cured. In Japanese and Chinese religions, as well, sandalwood is cherished and is the most common incense burned in worship and ritual.

Although sandalwood isn't widely used in food, the fruit, kernels, and nuts of Australian sandalwoods are foraged and eaten by the Aborigines.

When it comes to medicine, sandalwood was particularly popular in traditional herbal medicine as an antiseptic and a skin support. It was also used internally for urogenital issues. Nowadays, it is commonly used in soap making and in aromatherapy and perfumery. In fact, in the late '90s, western Australia saw a renewed interest in the oil and, at its peak, produced over 44,000 pounds of the stuff per year up until 2009. The oil was most commonly used in European fragrance industries up until that point and, thereafter, a large chunk of this production is used in India's chewing tobacco industry.

In India, sandalwood is also used in the cosmetic industry and, in fragrances, it is known to be a fixative, which means it extends the longevity and enhances the scent of the fragrances with which it's been blended.

Chemical Components

To generate the essential oil from sandalwood, the wood must be steam distilled. This results in the oil's key chemical components, which are primarily santyl acetate, beta santalol, and santalenes.

Main Properties of Sandalwood Essential Oil

Along with the properties previously mentioned in the introduction, sandalwood oil possesses antioxidant, anti-inflammatory, antibacterial, antifungal, antiviral, antiseptic, antispasmodic, antidepressant, aphrodisiac, astringent, sedative, diuretic, hypotensive, carminative, expectorant, digestive, tonic, and stimulant properties. With such a versatile range, sandalwood is well equipped to fight off any pathogen in the body's path.

Sandalwood, as mentioned, is composed of santyl acetate, beta santalol, and santalenes. These components are what instill the enormously beneficial properties within sandalwood essential oil. We'll outline these properties below.

Antioxidant

Anything high in antioxidants – whether fruit, beans, or essential oils – is a powerful advocate for your body. Antioxidants both protect against free radicals and repair their damage. What are free radicals? Free radicals are destructive chemicals that invade your body, produced by substances both inside and out. Some free radicals (or oxidants) form through normal bodily reactions, like inflammation, metabolism and aerobic respiration. Other free radicals form outside the body, but enter it due to exposure. These include harmful pollutants, toxins, smoking, alcohol, X-rays, and UV rays, to name a few. Although our bodies produce their own antioxidants, these often become damaged as we grow older; thus, introducing antioxidants into our bodies allows these nutrients and enzymes to assist in chemical reactions which destroy the oxidants or free radicals. Sandalwood essential oil is a moderate antioxidant, aiming to detox the body of free radicals that lead to disease.

Anti-inflammatory

External or internal inflammation can be reduced using sandalwood essential oil. For instance, if you or your patient has swollen fingers from arthritis or a swollen knee from a sport's injury, oral application of sandalwood essential oil may decrease irritation or redness, while also soothing the pain that accompanies inflammation.

Antifungal

While bacteria and viruses are plenty evil, fungi commonly lead to the deadliest infections, whether external or internal. Your ears, throat and nose are the most likely to become infected by fungi, the infections of which can be both excruciating and unsightly. If left untreated, fungal infections can kill, as they may spread to the brain. Sandalwood essential oil protects against these infections and more and is particularly effective against skin infections.

Antiviral

The antiviral protection that sandalwood essential oil grants will empower the immune system at its core, building up a tougher wall of security that most colds, measles or mumps are unlikely to scale. By boosting white blood cell count and function, this immune stimulant will ensure that your body is better prepared to protect against deadly viral infections.

Antibacterial

Sandalwood's antibacterial properties make it a powerful protectant against diseases produced by bacteria, such as oral and digestive bacterial infections. What's great is that, unlike some prescription drugs, sandalwood has no ill effects on bodily wellness or on the healthy natural flora that exists within the stomach and intestines.

Antiseptic

The antiseptic properties of sandalwood essential oil can be reaped topically, applied directly to wounds, or even through burning; the smoke from the oil may help destroy airborne germs. Internal use will help keep the wounds from becoming infections, while external use will support the body's natural function in inhibiting tetanus.

Antispasmodic

The antispasmodic properties of sandalwood essential

oil make it beneficial to such wellness issues as chronic coughing and other respiratory conditions, along with surgical processes, such as colonoscopy and gastroscopy.

Antidepressant

When it comes to psychological issues, the uplifting scent of sandalwood combats negative thoughts and, thereby, depression.

Aphrodisiac

As an aphrodisiac, sandalwood can help stimulate sexual arousal, thereby overriding impotence, frigidity, low libido, and erectile dysfunction.

Astringent

For those who do not know what an astringent is, it's a chemical compound that shrinks body tissues, which means it can aid skin issues and irritations, everything from acne to insect bites. The astringent property of sandalwood essential oil benefits everything from skin to hair to gums to muscles to intestines. As an astringent, sandalwood is an anti-agent, combating muscle loss through the ability to strengthen. This astringent and coagulant properties also mean that diarrhea can be relieved through use of sandalwood essential oil, as well as wound and cut bleeding.

Sedative

As a sedative, sandalwood sedates and calms by reducing anxiety, excitement or irritability. Though sedatives, alone, do not alleviate pain, they do calm the patient, making them less stressed and more compliant.

Diuretic

If you're looking to lose water weight and reduce blood pressure, sandalwood essential oil is your agent. The oil stimulates urination, promoting not only the loss of water weight, but the loss of fats, uric acid, sodium, and other body toxins.

Hypotensive

By supporting the relaxation of veins and arteries, sandalwood effectively reduces blood pressure. This boosts circulation and oxygenation to the organ systems and muscles, improving their function, as well as your metabolism, while also reducing the body's vulnerability to such risks as stroke, heart attack, brain hemorrhaging, or atherosclerosis.

Carminative

By supporting the reduction of excess gas buildup and/or removal of gas from the intestines, sandalwood essential oil provides relief from abdominal pain, excess sweating, and uncomfortable indigestion.

Expectorant

Throat or respiratory infections can be relieved using sandalwood essential oil. Acting as an expectorant, sandalwood breaks up and helps destroy the phlegm and mucus buildup that accompanies sinuses or respiratory infections. Inflamed throat and lungs – and, thus, coughing – can also be alleviated through the application of this oil.

Tonic

Sandalwood essential oil benefits each of the body's systems, whether nervous, digestive, respiratory or excretory, making it an unbeatable general tonic. The oil also supports the immune system by helping the body absorb nutrients.

Stimulant

Stimulants are often referred to as "uppers." This is because they produce mental or physical improvements or temporary enhancements of your bodily functions. For instance, you may grow more alert and awake or quicker on your feet after using a stimulant. Sandalwood essential oil can provide this temporary boost in mental and physical function, especially when it comes to the immune system.

Common Therapeutic Uses

Traditionally used to enhance the body's defenses against skin issues, sandalwood essential oil remains a significant skin support, protecting against several conditions, like scars, spots, and skin aging. Sandalwood essential oil supports overall wellness, while improving concentration and memory. Let's take a closer look at the common uses for this oil.

Immune System Booster

Sandalwood is a superb immune system support which boosts circulation and increases white blood cell count. The oil is akin to an immune shield braced to fight off inflammatory or fungal strains that attack the immune system. With such strong armor, this immune stimulant will ensure that your body is better prepared to protect against deadly infections.

Digestion

As a digestive aid, sandalwood essential oil's collective properties stimulate digestive enzyme secretion which serves to support issues like flatulence and stomach cramps.

Cardiovascular Wellness

Cardiovascular wellness can be maintained using sandalwood essential oil, which helps to reduce bad cholesterol (LDL) and boost good cholesterol (HDL). The oil's antioxidant properties and its ability to facilitate the dissolution of cholesterol that accumulates in arteries will help protect against cardiovascular issues, like heart disease or atherosclerosis.

Skin Care

Sandalwood essential oil supports the body's defenses against acne, wrinkles, dryness, and other skin issues. The oil's properties invigorate dull skin, while cleansing and eliminating excess oil. Whether using sandalwood essential oil to defy skin aging or to reduce adolescent skin issues, like pimples and acne, the antiseptic and astringent properties will enhance skin wellness at any age.

Weight Loss

Those who need an extra boost to lose unwanted body fat can pop a sandalwood capsule, which has been shown to suppress appetite and stimulate fat burn. The oil also helps stimulate and sustain energy, which means it can combat the lethargy and fatigue associated with unhealthy weight management.

Brain Stimulant

Sandalwood essential oil provides a refreshing and stimulating aroma that can relieve exhaustion and fatigue. It also produces mental focus and clarity, which is great when it comes to cognitive tasks, like studying or other brainwork.

Safety Precautions & Common Applications

Safety

Certain adverse effects may evolve when using pure essential oils. Some essential oils should not be used when pregnant, for example, as they may cause miscarriage. Allergic reactions, too, may occur, especially when applied topically. Always administer an allergy test before committing fully to topical application. When used with other medications, essential oils may react negatively. If you are on any current prescription medications or have a chronic illness, such as high blood pressure, epilepsy or liver disease, then researching the effects of essential oils against your own personal medical history will eliminate any potentially problematic issues.

Sandalwood has been approved by the FDA for internal consumption and so can be used as a dietary supplement. If you are pregnant, use with caution and at the discretion of your physician. If you have sensitive skin, test before extensive use and dilute accordingly. Otherwise, use neat or dilute 1:1 with a carrier oil. You can apply topically, diffuse or use as a dietary supplement.

Blends

Oftentimes, essential oils are manufactured as blends of several pure oils. For instance, the Protective Blend of certain brands is a mix of cinnamon, clove, rosemary, and eucalyptus. This blend can be used to boost the immune system to help support colds, viruses and flus. The downside to blends is that the more oils added to the mix, the higher the probability your patient may react negatively to the blend if he/she is prone to allergies. There is also the possibility of phototoxicity when working with blends, particularly if they include citrus oils. Be sure to read your labels before administering.

Regardless of these possible effects, essential oils are a viable option for supporting several conditions. Those looking to support or maintain their own personal wellness, or that of their families', should become educated on the uses of essential oils, their natural remedies and the methods of application. Only then can you begin building your kit of essential oils for survival.

Chapter 2 – Recipes for Sandalwood Essential Oil

In this chapter, we'll offer various recipes for sandalwood essential oil, both for pure sandalwood applications and blends. For pure applications, we've provided the appropriate dosage and method of administration to support specific ailments, from acne to wrinkles. When it comes to blends, herbalists and aromatherapists often combine sandalwood essential oil with ylang ylang, bergamot, vetiver, black pepper, rose, geranium, myrrh, and lavender. We'll offer some fantastic blending options in the second half of this chapter.

Pure Applications

Acne

Enhance your body's natural ability to clear acne by

diluting 2 drops of sandalwood essential oil in 4-5 drops of coconut oil and applying the combo to the affected area twice daily. Suggested application is before and after showering.

Alzheimer's Disease

Support the symptoms of Alzheimer's Disease by using neat or diluting sandalwood essential oil in a 1:1 ratio with a carrier oil; then apply topically, massaging into the base of the neck, the forehead, and the reflex points of the feet multiple times daily.

Anxiety

To relieve anxiety, place one drop of sandalwood essential oil into your palm and rub your hands together. Place your hand over your nose and mouth and inhale. You can also diffuse throughout your home to alleviate tension and stress, or apply two drops neat or diluted in a 1:1 ratio over the area of the heart and the back of the neck.

Aphrodisiac

Sandalwood has long been used to stimulate the libido. Diffuse regularly or apply topically, using neat or diluted in a 1:1 ratio with a carrier oil and massaging into the back of the neck and soles of the feet.

Pain

General pain can be eased by using neat or diluting sandalwood essential oil in a 1:1 ratio with a carrier oil; then apply topically, massaging over the respective reflex points of the feet in relation to the area of bodily pain or directly into the affected area.

Calming

Calm anger, stress or nerves by diffusing sandalwood essential oil throughout the home. You can also inhale directly or use neat or diluted in a 1:1 ratio with a carrier oil and apply topically in a full-body massage. Additionally, place one drop of the oil into your palm and rub your hands together. Place your hand over your nose and mouth and inhale.

Cancer

Help strengthen the body's natural defenses against cancer by using neat or diluting sandalwood essential oil in a 1:1 ratio with a carrier oil; then apply topically, massaging into the reflex points of the feet or over the affected area. You can also diffuse throughout the home for overall wellness.

Cartilage Injury

To relieve cartilage injuries, use neat or dilute sandalwood essential oil in a 1:1 ratio with a carrier oil and massage over the affected area or into the reflex points of the feet multiple times daily, until the injury clears up.

Confusion

Relieve confusion by applying a single drop of sandalwood across the brow.

Cramps

Alleviate menstrual, intestinal, or abdominal cramps by using neat or diluting sandalwood essential oil in a 1:1 ratio with a carrier oil and applying topically. Massage into the lower abdomen and back and into the reflex points of the feet.

Dandruff

As an antifungal, sandalwood essential oil balances the skin's pH levels and soothes dryness and irritation. Eliminate dandruff by applying directly to the scalp or add a drop or two to your shampoo and use as normal.

Depression

Combat depression by placing a drop of sandalwood essential oil on your pillow. You can also diffuse throughout the room or use the oil neat or diluted in a 1:1 ratio with a carrier oil and apply topically, massaging into scalp, neck and shoulders.

Fatigue

Combat fatigue by diffusing sandalwood essential oil or adding a few drops to your bathwater. You can also place a drop of oil into your hands, rub your palms together, cup them over your nose, and breathe deeply in and out for several minutes. And, lastly, you can use the oil neat or diluted in a 1:1 ratio with a carrier oil and apply in a full body massage or over your chest, the back of the neck, and the forehead. The oil will increase blood circulation, which will boost energy and brain function.

Fear

To help eliminate unwarranted fear, dilute sandalwood essential oil in a 1:1 ratio with a carrier oil and apply topically, massaging over the solar plexus and the heart. You can also administer aromatically, diffusing throughout the home or inhaling directly from the bottle.

Hair

For damaged or dry hair, place 1 or 2 drops of sandalwood essential oil in your daily shampoo and use as normal.

Hiccups

Rid of hiccups by massaging a drop of sandalwood essential oil over the throat and chest when they're in progress.

Insect Repellant

Repel pesky insects by using neat or diluting sandalwood essential oil in a 1:1 ratio with a carrier oil and applying topically to the skin. You can also diffuse throughout the home or place a drop on a cotton ball and set in any problem areas.

Insomnia

With its calming and relaxing scent, sandalwood essential oil can combat insomnia and ease you into a dreamless sleep. Use neat or dilute sandalwood essential oil in a 1:1 ratio with a carrier oil and massage into the reflex points of the feet, the forehead, and the back of the neck to trigger nervous system response. You might also diffuse or place a couple drops on your pillow or sheets.

Laryngitis

Relieve laryngitis by using neat or diluting sandalwood essential oil in a 1:1 ratio with a carrier oil and massaging over the throat multiple times daily. You can also add a drop to a warm water gargle.

Libido

Sandalwood has long been used to stimulate the libido. Diffuse regularly or use neat or diluted in a 1:1 ratio with a carrier oil and apply topically to the soles of the feet, the back of the neck, and over the pituitary gland.

Lou Gehrig's

To help relieve the symptoms of Lou Gehrig's disease, use sandalwood essential oil neat or diluted in a 1:1 ratio with a carrier oil and apply topically, massaging into the back of the neck, the forehead, and the reflex points multiple times daily.

Multiple Sclerosis

Soothe multiple sclerosis with a massage. Use neat or dilute sandalwood essential oil in a 1:1 ratio with a carrier oil and apply topically over the entire body or the soles of the feet. You may also diffuse or steam two drops of sandalwood essential oil in a pan of water then remove the steaming pan from the stove, pour into a bowl, place a towel over your head and inhale.

Rashes

Rashes can be alleviated by using neat sandalwood essential oil or diluted in a 1:1 ratio with a carrier oil and apply topically to the affected area. The oil will reduce itching and protect against infection while accelerating support.

Skin (Chapped, Dry, Cracked, Sensitive, Eczema, Acne, Dermatitis, etc.)

Sandalwood essential oil can support all types of skin conditions. Use sandalwood essential oil neat or dilute in a

1:1 ratio with a carrier oil and apply topically to the affected area. You can also add a drop of sandalwood to your daily skin regimen.

Stress

Combat stress by steaming two drops of sandalwood essential oil in a pan of water, remove the steaming pan from the stove, pour into a bowl, place a towel over your head and inhale. If you don't feel it's done its job the first time, you can reheat that same water and use it once more without adding more oil. You can also place a drop onto your shirt collar for portable stress relief, diffuse in the home, or apply topically to the chest, the top of the head, and the reflex points of the feet.

Tumors

To protect against tumors or reduce their growth, use sandalwood essential oil neat or dilute in a 1:1 ratio with a carrier oil and apply topically to the affected area or into the reflex points of the feet multiple times daily. Be sure, of course, to consult your physician beforehand.

Ulcer

Target ulcers externally by using neat or diluting sandalwood essential oil in a 1:1 ratio with a carrier oil and applying topically, massaging into the stomach, the affected area, and into the reflex points of the feet.

Vitiligo

Massage 1-2 drops over the areas of concern 1-2 times a day.

Wounds

Enhance wound wellness by adding a few drops of sandalwood essential oil to a spray bottle filled with distilled water. Spray over the wound. You may also apply a few drops to a spritz bath and soak the wound for 10-15 minutes. Additionally, you may use neat or dilute sandalwood in a 1:1 ratio with a carrier oil and apply topically to the affected area.

Wrinkles

Protect against wrinkles or reduce their appearance by using sandalwood essential oil neat or diluting in a 1:1 ratio with a carrier oil and massaging over the affected area. You can also add a drop or two to your daily skincare regimen. Be careful around the eyes.

Blends

Anti-Aging Salve

Ingredients

- 5 drops Geranium Essential Oil
- 5 drops Frankincense Essential Oil
- 5 drops Myrrh Essential Oil
- 5 drops Rosemary Essential Oil
- 5 drops Lemon Essential Oil
- 10 drops Rosehip Essential Oil
- 10 drops Carrot Seed Essential Oil
- 10 drops Sandalwood Essential Oil
- ½ cup Apricot Kernel Oil

Directions

To reduce the signs of skin aging, combine all ingredients in a small glass jar or container, blending well. After your evening facial routine, apply to areas of concern. Use as needed, blending well before each use.

Aphrodisiac Massage Blend

Ingredients

- 1 drop Ginger Essential Oil
- 1 drop Clove Essential Oil
- 2 drops Cinnamon Essential Oil
- 2 drops Peppermint Essential Oil
- 3 drops Jasmine Essential Oil
- 3 drops Vanilla Absolute
- 2 ounces Carrier Oil

Directions

To stimulate sexual arousal for men and women, combine all ingredients in a small bowl, blending well. Apply in a full body massage or into the reflex points (*caution: cinnamon essential oil is hot and may irritate sensitive skin; if you are prone to skin irritation, increase the amount of carrier oil).

Aphrodisiac Massage Blend II

Ingredients

- 2 drops Black Pepper Essential Oil
- 2 drops Ginger Essential Oil
- 3 drops Wild Orange Essential Oil
- 3 drops Rosemary Essential Oil
- 4 drops Ylang Ylang Essential Oil
- 4 drops Bergamot Essential Oil
- 4 drops Sandalwood Essential Oil
- 4 ounces Carrier Oil (fractionated coconut oil recommended)

Directions

To stimulate sexual arousal for men and women, combine all ingredients in a small bowl, blending well. Apply in a full body massage or into the reflex points. Store in a glass bottle.

Aphrodisiac Massage Oil for Men

Ingredients

- 2 drops Patchouli Essential Oil
- 3 drops Peppermint Essential Oil
- 3 drops Ginger Essential Oil
- 4 drops Cedarwood Essential Oil
- 4 drops Sandalwood Essential Oil
- 4 drops Lavender Essential Oil
- 2 Ounces Carrier Oil

Directions

To stimulate sexual arousal for men, combine all ingredients in a small bowl, blending well. Apply in a full body massage or into the reflex points.

Aphrodisiac Massage Oil for Women

Ingredients

- 2 drops Patchouli Essential Oil
- 3 drops Rose Essential Oil
- 3 drops Vanilla Absolute
- 3 drops Sandalwood Essential Oil
- 4 drops Jasmine Essential Oil
- 4 drops Ylang Ylang Essential Oil
- 2 Ounces Carrier Oil

Directions

To stimulate sexual arousal for women, combine all ingredients in a small bowl, blending well. Apply in a full body massage or into the reflex points.

Aphrodisiac Perfume

Ingredients

- 2 drops Vanilla Essential Oil
- 3 drops Sandalwood Essential Oil
- 3 drops Cedarwood Essential Oil
- 300 mL 70% Grain Alcohol or Vodka (no rubbing alcohol)

Directions

To create an aphrodisiac perfume, combine all ingredients in a perfume bottle and shake well. Let sit for a week, for the ingredients to synergize and set. Use as normal.

Brain Stimulant

Ingredients

- 30 drops Balsam Fir Essential Oil
- 15 drops Sandalwood Essential Oil
- 15 drops Frankincense Essential Oil
- 8 drops Helichrysum Essential oil
- 3 drops Melissa Essential Oil
- 2 drops Peppermint Essential Oil
- 1 ounce Carrier Oil

Directions

To help stimulate the brain, combine all ingredients in a small glass bottle or container and blend well. When needed, apply 10-12 drops of the blend per ounce of carrier oil and massage into the temples, forehead, back of the neck, and into the reflex points of the feet.

Brittle or Damaged Hair

Ingredients

- 15 drops Sandalwood Essential Oil
- 10 drops Lavender Essential Oil
- 5 drops Geranium Essential Oil
- 1 ounce Jojoba Oil

Directions

To repair damaged or brittle hair, mix all ingredients in a small container until well combined. Massage into dry hair, place a shower cap over your head, and let sit for 20-30 minutes. Wash hair twice with shampoo to remove excess oil.

Creative Stimulant

Ingredients

- 1 drop Lime Essential Oil
- 1 drop Clary Sage Essential Oil
- 1 drop Sandalwood Essential Oil
- 3 drops Carrier Oil

Directions

To stimulate creativity, combine ingredients in a small glass container and apply topically to your pulse points.

Erectile Dysfunction Blend

Ingredients

- 1 drop Jasmine Essential Oil
- 1 drop Black Pepper Essential Oil
- 1 drop Sandalwood Essential Oil
- 1 drop Nutmeg Essential Oil
- 1 drop Ginger Essential Oil
- 1 Tbsp. Sweet Almond Oil

Directions

The issue of erectile dysfunction is often influenced by poor blood flow. The oils in this blend enhance blood flow and circulation. To administer, you may apply to a warm compress or massage into the lower back. You can also add the oils (no need for the carrier oil) to a hot bath.

Facial Blend

Ingredients

- 4 drops Neroli Essential Oil
- 2 drops Lavender Essential Oil
- 2 drops Sandalwood Essential Oil
- 1 drop Geranium Essential Oil
- 1 drop Ylang Ylang Essential Oil
- ½ ounce Almond Oil
- ½ ounce Rosehip Oil

Directions

For a fresh facial blend, mix all ingredients in a small jar or container until well combined. Massage in a circular motion into the face, avoiding the eyes. Use as needed as a substitute for your daily moisturizer.

Fatigue

Ingredients

- 1 drop Ginger Essential Oil
- 2 drops Clary Sage Essential Oil
- 2 drops Sandalwood Essential Oil
- 2 drops Cilantro Essential Oil
- 3 drops Frankincense Essential Oil
- ½ Tbsp. Carrier Oil

Directions

To combat fatigue, combine all ingredients in a small bowl or container, blending well. Apply topically to the forearms and the back of the neck, inhaling the scent deeply.

Ligament/Tendon Injury Regeneration

Ingredients

- 10 drops Marjoram Essential Oil
- 10 drops Lemongrass Essential Oil
- 5 drops Lavender Essential Oil
- 5 drops Sandalwood Essential Oil
- 5 drops Cypress Essential Oil
- 1 tsp Carrier Oil

Directions

For a regenerative blend after tendon or ligament injury, combine the essential oils in a roller bottle for easy application, topping up with a carrier oil. To administer, apply directly from the roller to the affected area and, if you have sensitive skin, add an additional teaspoon of carrier oil to the application.

Relaxing Diffusion Blend

Ingredients

- 2 drops Sandalwood Essential Oil
- 4 drops Ginger Essential Oil
- 6 drops Lime Essential Oil
- 6 drops Grapefruit Essential Oil
- 6 drops Bergamot Essential Oil

Directions

In a small jar or container, mix all ingredients until well combined. Diffuse several drops of the blend as needed, especially during stressful times or when you want to unwind.

Scar Salve

Ingredients

- 2 drops Sandalwood Essential Oil
- 4 drops Lavender Essential Oil
- 6 drops Helichrysum Essential Oil
- 6 drops Myrrh Essential Oil
- 1 Tbsp. Grapeseed Oil

Directions

To fade the appearance of scars or protect against scarring, combine all ingredients in a small glass bowl or container, blending well. Apply topically to affected area.

Snoring Relief & Sleep Stimulant

Ingredients

- 4 drops Marjoram Essential Oil
- 4 drops Sandalwood Essential Oil
- 4 drops Lemongrass Essential Oil
- 2 drops Lavender Essential Oil
- 2 drops Myrtle Essential Oil
- ¼ cup Sweet Almond Oil

Directions

To relieve the snoring and induce sleep, combine all ingredients in a small bowl, blending well. Apply topically, massaging into the reflex points of the feet and over the body.

Warming Massage Blend

Ingredients

- 2 drops Ginger Essential Oil
- 3 drops Black Pepper Essential Oil
- 5 drops Sandalwood Essential Oil
- 15 drops Ylang Ylang Essential Oil
- 15 mL Carrier Oil

Directions

In a small bowl or container, mix all ingredients until well combined. Warm slightly then to help relax and relieve sore muscles and stimulate libido, apply in a full-body massage.

Chapter 3 – Sandalwood Essential Oil Studies

Many studies have been done on essential oils to uncover and prove their therapeutic qualities. In the case of the great number of sandalwood studies, many of the properties attributed to the essential oil (noted in this book and elsewhere) are quite often validated through the research from accredited universities and published by reputable scientific journals. In this chapter, we'll discuss a small portion of these studies. It's important to note that our knowledge of essential oils is constantly evolving. Keep up with any recent research, as it may turn up even further valuable uses for these miracle oils.

Study 1 – Herpes Simplex

In this study published by *Antimicrobial Agents & Chemotherapy*, the activities of sandalwood essential oil on herpes simplex virus were examined, with the following results: "Acyclovir-resistant clinical isolates of herpes simplex virus type 1 (HSV-1) were analyzed in vitro for their susceptibilities to essential oils of ginger, thyme, hyssop, and sandalwood. All essential oils exhibited high levels of viricidal activity against acyclovir-sensitive strain KOS and acyclovir-resistant HSV-1 clinical isolates and reduced plaque formation significantly."

This study demonstrated sandalwood oil's antiviral activity regarding Herpes Simplex virus. According to the demonstrated activity of the oils, the mechanism by which they inhibit the virus is through interfering with virion envelope structures. These structures are necessary for the virus to enter host cells. This demonstrated antiviral activity indicates the efficacy of sandalwood essential oil in supporting the body's defenses against Herpes Simplex virus.

Reference
http://www.ncbi.nlm.nih.gov/pubmed/17353250]
http://www.ncbi.nlm.nih.gov/pmc/articles/PMC1855548/

Study 2 – Antibacterial Properties

In this study published by *Evidence-Based Complementary and Alternative Medicine*, the antibacterial effects of sandalwood essential oil were examined, with the following results: "Hospital-acquired infections and antibiotic-resistant bacteria continue to be major wellness concerns worldwide. Particularly problematic is methicillin-resistant Staphylococcus aureus (MRSA) and its ability to cause severe soft tissue, bone or implant infections…Several common and hospital-acquired bacterial and yeast isolates (6 Staphylococcus strains including MRSA, 4 Streptococcus strains and 3 Candida strains including Candida krusei) were tested for their susceptibility for Eucalyptus, Tea tree, Thyme white, Lavender, Lemon, Lemongrass, Cinnamon, Grapefruit, Clove Bud, Sandalwood, Peppermint, Kunzea and Sage oil with the agar diffusion test. Olive oil, Paraffin oil, Ethanol (70%), Povidone iodine, Chlorhexidine and hydrogen peroxide (H(2) O(2)) served as controls. Large prevailing effective zones of inhibition were observed for Thyme white, Lemon, Lemongrass and Cinnamon oil. The other oils also showed considerable efficacy. Remarkably, almost all tested oils demonstrated efficacy against hospital-acquired isolates and reference strains, whereas Olive and Paraffin oil from the control group produced no inhibition. As proven in vitro, essential oils represent a cheap and effective antiseptic topical treatment option even for antibiotic-resistant strains as MRSA and antimycotic-resistant Candida species."

S. aureus is Gram-positive bacterium. Methicillin-resistant Staphylococcus aureus (MRSA) is any strain of S. aureus that's naturally developed a resistance to antibiotics, including penicillin. This hospital-acquired infection is now limitedly endemic. Being resistant to standard medications, these strains – although not more virulent than other S. aureus strains – may result in infections that are tough to treat. Hospitals, nursing homes, and prisons largely house MRSA, and patients with weak immune systems and open wounds are most at risk.

The study found that sandalwood essential oil had an inhibitory effect on MRSA strains, as well as several Streptococcus and Candida strains tested, without any cytotoxic effect on skin cells. These results indicate that sandalwood essential oil could potentially be used as an antibacterial agent for this strain of bacteria.

Reference

http://www.ncbi.nlm.nih.gov/pubmed/19473851]

Study 3 – Insecticidal Properties

In this study available on PubMed, the insecticidal activities of sandalwood essential oil were examined, with the following results: "Mosquitoes in the larval stage are attractive targets for pesticides because mosquitoes breed in water, and thus, it is easy to deal with them in this habitat. The use of conventional pesticides in the water sources, however, introduces many risks to people and/or the environment. Natural pesticides, especially those derived from plants, are more promising in this aspect. Aromatic plants and their essential oils are very important sources of many compounds that are used in different respects. In this study, the oils of 41 plants were evaluated for their effects against third-instar larvae of Aedes aegypti, Anopheles stephensi and Culex quinquefasciatus…Thirteen oils from 41 plants (camphor, thyme, amyris, lemon, cedarwood, frankincense, dill, myrtle, juniper, black pepper, verbena, helichrysum and sandalwood) induced 100% mortality after 24 h, or even after shorter periods."

Prevalent primarily in the tropics, dengue fever affects between 50 and 528 million people annually and is endemic in over 110 countries. The infection is transmitted via mosquitoes which carry the dengue virus, among them the Ae. aegypti species. The resulting symptoms of the viral disease include joint and muscle pain, fever, and skin rash which is akin to the measles. The disease can sometimes escalate into dengue hemorrhagic fever or dengue shock syndrome, each far more fatal than common dengue fever.

There is no commercial vaccine for dengue fever, therefore eliminating the mosquitoes' habitats and reducing exposure to bites is the primary preventative measure. Treatment of dengue fever, as well, is supported primarily through rehydration with no pharmaceutical medication yet developed to target the virus directly (although medications are in development).

Culex quinquefasciatus and Anopheles stephensi are malaria-carrying mosquitoes, while the former is also known to transmit West Nile virus. West Nile virus was first discovered in Africa, but now affects all corners of the world, including the continental United States, with 286 deaths in 2012, alone. Symptoms of West Nile may include fever, fatigue, headaches, muscle aches, nausea, vomiting, rash, malaise, and anorexia. Most of the global malarial infections are in Africa, with over 247 million human infections to date, worldwide, 98% of which occur in Africa. Malarial symptoms include nausea, vomiting, fatigue, headache, chills, sweats, and fever.

According to this study, sandalwood essential oil shows promise in the terminating of the virus-carrying mosquito larvae. The oil demonstrated 100% mortality after 24 hours against Aedes aegypti, making it an effective potential mosquito control in areas where dengue fever, malaria, or West Nile are endemic.

Reference
http://www.ncbi.nlm.nih.gov/pubmed/16642386]

Study 4 – Anticancer Properties

In this study published in *Chinese Medicine*, the anticancer activities of sandalwood essential oil were examined, with the following results: "Frankincense (Boswellia carterii, known as Ru Xiang in Chinese) and sandalwood (Santalum album, known as Tan Xiang in Chinese) are cancer preventive and therapeutic agents in Chinese medicine. Their biologically active ingredients are usually extracted from frankincense by hydro distillation and sandalwood by distillation. This study aims to investigate the anti-proliferative and pro-apoptotic activities of frankincense and sandalwood essential oils in cultured human bladder cancer cells…The effects of frankincense and sandalwood essential oils on J82 cells and UROtsa cells involved different mechanisms leading to cancer cell death. While frankincense essential oil elicited selective cancer cell death via NRF-2-mediated oxidative stress, sandalwood essential oil induced non-selective cell death via DNA damage and cell cycle arrest."

Bladder cancer occurs in the epithelial lining of the urinary bladder, with around 77% of those diagnosed in America surviving past five years. However, with around 430,000 fresh diagnoses and 165,000 deaths annually, bladder cancer clocks in as the 9th leading cause of cancer, making it a target for progressive studies.

Sandalwood essential oil was tested on bladder cancer cells to evaluate the oil's anti-proliferative and pro-apoptotic activities, particularly when compared to those of frankincense. The results revealed that sandalwood essential oil induced apoptosis, or programmed cell death, which demonstrates the part sandalwood may play in the cytotoxicity of cancer cells.

Reference
http://www.ncbi.nlm.nih.gov/pubmed/25006348]

http://www.ncbi.nlm.nih.gov/pmc/articles/PMC4086286/pdf/1749-8546-9-18.pdf]

Study 5 – Anti-inflammatory Properties

In this study available on PubMed, the anti-inflammatory effects of sandalwood essential oil were examined, with the following results: "Medicinally, sandalwood oil (SO) has been attributed with anti-inflammatory properties; however, mechanism(s) for this activity have not been elucidated. To examine how SOs affect inflammation, cytokine antibody arrays and enzyme-linked immunosorbent assays were used to assess changes in production of cytokines and chemokines by co-cultured human dermal fibroblasts and neo-epidermal keratinocytes exposed to lipopolysaccharides and SOs from Western Australian and East Indian sandalwood trees or to the primary SO components, α-santalol and β-santalol...The ability of SOs to mimic ibuprofen non-steroidal anti-inflammatory drugs that act by inhibiting cyclooxygenases suggests a possible mechanism for the observed anti-inflammatory properties of topically applied SOs and provides a rationale for use in products requiring anti-inflammatory effects."

The objective of this study was to evaluate the anti-inflammatory effects of sandalwood essential oil. In the study, sandalwood essential oils were shone to suppress the cytokines and chemokines, which result in inflammation due to oxidative stress. These results demonstrate the mechanism by which sandalwood essential oil inhibits inflammation, thereby suggesting its efficacy in use as an anti-inflammatory on its own or in anti-inflammatory products.

Reference
http://www.ncbi.nlm.nih.gov/pubmed/24318647]

Study 6 – Malaria

In this study available on PubMed, sandalwood essential oil's effects on malaria were examined, with the following results: "The anti-plasmodial activity of 47 essential oils and 10 of their constituents were screened for in vitro activity against Plasmodium falciparum. Five of these essential oils (sandalwood, caraway, monarda, nutmeg, and Thujopsis dolabrata var. hondai) and 2 constituents (thymoquinone and hinokitiol) were found to be active against P. falciparum in vitro, with 50% inhibitory concentration (IC50) values equal to or less than 1.0 microg/ml."

This study tested sandalwood essential oil, along with other essential oils, against Plasmodium falciparum. Plasmodium falciparum is a parasite that is transmitted through a mosquito and can cause the most dangerous strain of malaria, with the highest mortality rate. In fact, almost every death due to malaria is caused by this parasite. The worldwide cases of malaria were at over 198 million in 2013, according to the World Health Organization. At 98% of the total, most of the global malarial infections are in Africa, and more than 75% of those infections are caused by P. falciparum. Malarial symptoms include nausea, vomiting, fatigue, headache, chills, sweats, and fever. This study found that sandalwood essential oil is active against the parasite, inhibiting 50% of P. falciparum at equal to or less than 1.0 microg/ml.

Reference & Photo Credit:
http://www.ncbi.nlm.nih.gov/pubmed/23082579]

Chapter 4 – The Ins & Outs of Essential Oils

Where do essential oils come from?

Plants and plant species naturally produce essential oils for various reasons, one being to draw pollinator insects to them, another being to repel invading organisms (bacteria, animals). Several chemical compounds compose each plant's essential oil, and the combination of these compounds are specific to each oil, which then instills in the oil its own unique properties. Essential oils can be harnessed from all sorts of plant components, including flowers, leaves, bark, fruit, roots, and resin. For instance, cinnamon oil is harnessed from bark, lemon oil from the peel, and lavender oil from lavender flowers. Certain plants can produce a few chemical variants of the same essential oil, which are acquired from different parts of the plant.

Some of these parts produce a large amount of oil, while others produce just a smidgen. The oil's quality and potency depends upon several factors, including the subspecies of the plant, its soil conditions, the time of year and even the time of day you harvest it.

How are essential oils extracted?

Essential oils can be extracted from plants through various methods, including pressing, distillation, solvent and maceration. Let's take a brief look at each:

Pressing Method

Commonly used with citrus fruit, the pressing method extracts the oil through a technique which involves pushing the fruit peels through a press. Oily fruits and plants are best suited for this technique. Orange oil, for example, is extracted from orange skins through the pressing method.

Distillation Method

This technique harkens back to the days of old-timey moonshiners, as the same sort of method used to create strong liquor can be used to extract essential oils. Using a still, boiled water and plant materials will create steam which is then cooled by coils and condensed into a combination of water and oil. This combination doesn't mix, so the oil can then be extracted from it.

Solvent Method

Through a multi-step process, certain plant and flower oils can be extracted using alcohol and other solvents, which extort the essential oil from the plant materials.

Maceration Method

When a "carrier" or fixed oil or lard is mixed with the plant material and set out in the sun, over a period, the carrier oil is infused with the plant's essence. Heat sources, other than the sun, are often used to speed the process. Throughout the process, more plant material is added to produce a more potent oil.

How do you use essential oils?

Although some studies about the effectiveness of essential oils are conducted by small companies or even individuals, several them are conducted by the food and cosmetic industries. In general, the pharmaceutical industry shows next to no interest in herbal medicine, primarily because there are few options to patent such products. Being as such, the product's lack of profitability results in a lack of research funding. Regardless, the historical uses of essential oils tell us what we need to know: these oils have been effectively administered for centuries. The therapeutic qualifications of essential oils can be plotted in the survival of humans across cultures and generations.

Another reason that studies on essential oils have not resulted in much conclusive evidence as to their overall effectiveness is because definitive results are sometimes difficult to prove, as the quality of each batch of oil can vary for several reasons. One is that essential oils are impossible to standardize. As mentioned above, even the slightest variance in soil conditions and the time of harvesting – as well as innumerable other factors – will produce a different product quality and potency. In addition, essential oils are often obtained from various species of the same plant; Eucalyptus radiata and Eucalyptus globulus can both be used in the making of therapeutic-grade eucalyptus oil and, as a result, they may have slightly different properties and degrees of strength or effectiveness.

Just as there are many methods by which to extract essential oils, there are several methods to administer them therapeutically. The variety of chemical compounds in each essential oil means that their benefits and applications also vary across the board. Below are a few of these methods.

Topical Administration

Direct application of many essential oils works like a sponge, as skin sops up chemicals and other things (like sunlight, for instance). Topical application is best when you want to clear up an ailment on the skin's surface or in the underlying muscle tissue. When applying topically, you may either massage the oil into the skin or simply dab on the skin for therapeutic results. You might combine the essential oil with a carrier oil for topical use to dilute its potency. This is safer, as the oil is so concentrated. You may support your body's defenses against rash or muscle pain in this manner, but you should always test your patient for allergens before applying. Adverse effects are produced by natural chemicals as much as synthetic ones; poison ivy, for example.

To test for allergens, place a drop or two on your patient's inner forearm. If a rash develops within 12 to 24 hours, then the patient is allergic. In addition, phototoxicity – sun exposure resulting in an exacerbated burn – may be an issue when citrus oils are applied topically. So, one must proceed with caution when applying essential oils using this method.

Inhalation Therapy

Commonly known as "aromatherapy", this essential oil application is effective for inner ailments, like sore throat or cold. In a steaming bowl of distilled or sterilized water, add a few drops of essential oil and, with a towel over your head, bend over the bowl and inhale. The towel captures the vapors, making the technique even more effective. Essential oils can also be placed in a diffuser or potpourri throughout a room to produce somewhat diluted therapeutic effects.

Ingestion

When using this method, proceed with caution. Direct ingestion of essential oils must be monitored and applied in small doses that are diluted in a tablespoon or more of any carrier oil – olive oil, for example. If you are unsure of dosage amounts, make a tea with the relevant herb instead. Although the effects of this diluted use may be weaker, this application is a better alternative than an overdose of essential oils.

What are the general benefits of using essential oils?

Replacement for Prescription Drugs

One practical benefit for using essential oils is, of course, their substitutive nature. Many believe that they can replace Rx drugs, which is the ultimate reason to educate yourself on their application and to begin stockpiling your essential oil supply. Although it is our opinion that 100% pure essential oils that carry no harmful side effects are better to support the body and its functions, we recommend that you consult your physician before replacing your prescription or over-the-counter medications.

One of the potential threats of economic or social collapse is the lack of resources, and primarily the inability to procure prescription drugs. Being as such, finding suitable alternatives should be a priority when prepping for the worst.

Their portability is also a major bonus when it comes to survival prepping. The fact that these ultra-concentrated oils take up little-to-no space makes toting them to your shelter all the simpler should the need arise. And, because essential oils are highly concentrated, the application used in most procedures requires only a drop or two of oil, which means that tiny bottle will be long-lasting (example 15mL bottle contains approx. 250 drops).

Cheap, but Effective Alternative

Though money may be the last thing on your mind when it comes to prepping for a survival situation (money may even be obsolete in the event of social collapse), it is worth noting that the expense of essential oils pales in comparison to prescription drugs. In fact, whether you are forced to survive on essential oils due to a lack of prescription reserves, in some cases, you might consider substituting your prescriptions for these inexpensive alternatives regardless. Essential oils are a cheap, but equally effective alternative to prescription medicine.

No Expiration Date

Another benefit of essential oils is that they do not expire, neither do they have "proper storage" requirements. Several medicines and therapeutic products must be replaced every couple years, so this sets essential oils ahead of the pack when it comes to shelf life.

Versatility

Essential oils also offer great versatility. Apart from providing wellness benefits, essential oils can be repurposed for household and hygienic applications. For instance, if you're looking for something that might serve your dental hygiene needs in a time of crisis, thieves oil is your go-to essential oil. If you want to maintain your skin's wellness, frankincense and lavender will do the trick; the latter also serves as sunscreen, so you can prevent sun damage as well.

When it comes to the house or shelter, you can use essential oils to deodorize, which will come in handy in a disaster scenario where things might start to smell fishy due to lack of proper utilities and care. For example, after the 2011 tsunami and the subsequent nuclear reactor meltdown in Japan, a nurse named Risa Nakahira used essential oils to deodorize and sanitize putrid public bathrooms in overpopulated evacuation facilities. As relief workers searched for survivors, often wading through debris and decay, Nakahira also deodorized their boots and masks using essential oils. The possibilities of these natural oils are endless.

They are also versatile when it comes to the range of patients they're capable of supporting. The wellness of everyone from your great grandfather to your infant baby can be fortified with the aid of essential oils in the appropriate dosage. They even come in handy when supporting livestock or pets. From teething infants to dementia in the elderly, from teenagers with acne to dogs with urinary tract infections, essential oils can serve any patient with nearly any ailment.

Conclusion

Now that you know all about what sandalwood essential oil can do for you – where it originates, how it's extracted, its benefits and properties, and the different methods of administration – you can use it confidently to support the body's defenses against wellness issues and start to assemble a kit of essential oils for survival.

The various benefits of essential oils and their properties are countless. To build your own kit, first focus on acquiring the essential oils which may bear more relevance to your wellness issues or the potential wellness threats within your environment. When it comes to fortifying the immune system, for instance, sandalwood essential oil will be one of your more crucial oils, due to its immune supportive properties.

Used as a supplement or as your go-to for inflammation, cardiovascular wellness, or skin care, the application of sandalwood essential oil in medicine has survived for centuries and will survive centuries more. When it comes down to it, you don't need to rely on pharmaceuticals; essential oils, herbs, and plenty of other natural ingredients can be used to help support any number of wellness issues, whether ailment or injury.

Essential oils are essential to your survival in the case of viral outbreak, social collapse or natural disaster because, when the SHTF, your access to pharmaceuticals will likely

either be limited or eliminated altogether. Alternatives to
our modern-day standard will equate survival when no
other option exists. And when it comes to a life-or-death
situation, you can't let your wellness decline, no matter the
state of the world.

DISCLAIMER AND/OR LEGAL NOTICES: Every effort has been made to accurately represent this book and it's potential. Results vary with every individual, and your results may or may not be different from those depicted. No promises, guarantees or warranties, whether stated or implied, have been made that you will produce any specific result from this book. Your efforts are individual and unique, and may vary from those shown. Your success depends on your efforts, background and motivation.

The material in this publication is provided for educational and informational purposes only and is not intended as medical advice. The information contained in this book should not be used to diagnose or treat any illness, metabolic disorder, disease or health problem. Always consult your physician or healthcare provider before beginning any nutrition or exercise program. Use of the programs, advice, and information contained in this book is at the sole choice and risk of the reader.